THE ELEPHANT IN THE ROOM

THE ELEPHANT IN THE ROOM

how to overcome your psychological barriers to weight loss success

Gemma Rayne Fountain

Exercise Physiologist, Integrative Nutrition Health Coach & Fitness Expert

Dedicated to Anne Quarles (Hughes), my 9th grade English teacher.

Thank you for paying attention.

1

Introduction

You know you should exercise. You know which foods are healthier than others. When out for dinner, you know you should order the salad but when the server asks you what you want, "A bacon double cheeseburger with fries" rushes out of your mouth before you even realize what happened. Deep down you know what you need to do to reach your health, fitness, weight loss and nutrition goals. Yet, as I'm sure you've learned, knowing and doing are two very different things.

With health, fitness, nutrition, and weight loss ads posted all over the TV, magazines, apps, and the web, you have an unlimited amount of resources at your fingertips. And yet, for some reason, you still can't stick to a program or maintain results.

It has become blatantly apparent that knowledge is not the issue.

How many diets have you tried believing, with each new fad, that *"this is the one"*? How many months of gym memberships have you paid for that have gone unused, hoping that tomorrow you'll wake up with motivation? How many fruits and veggies have turned brown and smelly in your refrigerator only to be tossed in the trash instead of included in your healthy way of eating? Maybe the next fad is the *magic bullet* to get you where you so deeply desire to be.

The truth is there is no 'magic bullet.' There is one, and only one, reason why you are not achieving success. That reason, is you.

You are the reason—and this is great news, because since it is you, you have control over your obstacle.

You have the power to effect change within yourself. You don't need permission to become a better you, however, you may need a little help.

I hope this book can be that help.

Chances are there is only one problem that is standing in your way to great success. There may be one, solitary issue preventing you from that health, fitness or weight loss goal. It could just be a single obstacle that you are not addressing, and that issue is...

The Elephant in the Room!

2

The Elephant in the Room Defined

If you look up the term *elephant in the room* on *Wikipedia, The Free Encyclopedia* online you'll find this:

> *"Elephant in the room"* is an English metaphorical idiom for an obvious truth that is either being ignored or going unaddressed.
>
> It is based on the idea that an elephant in a room would be impossible to overlook; thus, people in the room who pretend the elephant is not there have chosen to avoid dealing with the looming issue.[i]

For years, I have watched fitness professionals and nutritional experts share all the tips and tricks to successful exercise and healthy eating. Throughout all these years, I have watched people work very hard only to quit, be defeated by lack of results, and self-sabotage success. I was one of these people for many years.

Knowledge of health and fitness is not the problem. We have long had immeasurable information on these topics. First, it was VHS tapes and healthy cook books, then it was DVDs and healthy cooking shows, and now we have the internet with YouTube, social media, and apps. There are so many resources for health, fitness, and weight loss; yet, as a nation, we are heavier and unhealthier than ever.

When I was new to the fitness industry, I knew that the training I received was lacking in the most important element of success—the psychological factor. I was giving my clients the greatest and simplest information for fitness and weight loss success, but very few clients reached their ultimate goals. Not only did I know all the right information, I was certified to train others, and yet I could not even reach my own fitness goals. I thought, "If I can't achieve fitness and weight loss success myself, who am I to teach others?" Not only did I feel like a hypocrite, I felt that I was letting my clients down. I knew that my nutrition and fitness knowledge on its own was not enough. We had to go deeper. Why weren't we sticking to a healthy diet? Why did we make choices we knew were bad for us? Why did we skip the gym? Why could we not stay motivated?

I knew these problems were psychological; however, I was taught that it was beyond my scope of practice to address such issues. That was for mental health professionals. I felt that I had failed as a fitness leader by continually ignoring the most important aspect of success. The number one reason why clients don't reach their goals—the most powerful part of the human body—is the brain.

I do not pretend to be a therapist, but I can certainly expose my observations. I can suggest to clients that they embark on a journey of healing with self-introspection, self-help books and/or therapy. I can let my clients know that it is completely acceptable to not be perfect, to acknowledge that imperfection, and to seek help to improve yourself. In fact, getting help is the fastest way to healing.

It's time to start a loving and open discussion about the mental obstacles which are preventing us from being our best in every area of our lives - including health, body image, fitness, and weight.

It is through my own journey and battling my own elephants in the room that I have found success and maintained it. The journey has not been quick nor easy, but I am a better and more successful person because of it.

It has been my mission to lovingly, openly, and with total acceptance discuss the psychological reasons why people do not achieve their goals with health, fitness, nutrition and weight loss (which, often times, also affect goals in all other areas of life).

Until you begin to attack, address and unravel your own psychological barriers to achievement, those self-imposed barriers to exercise and weight loss triumph, you are fighting an uphill battle with very little hope for maintained success. It's time to get your brooms out folks. We're cleaning out your emotional cupboard!

3

You Are a Beautiful and
Unique Snowflake

I have been a fitness professional since 1999. During my years of training clients one-on-one and in small group settings, teaching fitness classes and health coaching, I have noticed a lot of things.

I have noticed that most people make the same mistakes when doing lunges and squats. I have noticed that most people do push-ups incorrectly. I have noticed that people, before starting a fitness program, often believe they are in better shape than they really are. I have noticed that people have the best intentions but don't always follow through. I have noticed that people are more likely to believe the far-fetched "quick-fix" baloney than proven, science-based information which gets results but requires work. I have noticed that people are willing to take pharmaceutical medications with laundry lists of side effects without question; yet, are apprehensive about taking a multi-vitamin with little to no adverse effects, which would likely improve their health and decrease their need for pharmaceuticals.

I have noticed that most people are the same and suffer from the same obstacles to success in the areas of fitness and weight loss. We aren't as different as you may want to think.

Many people, after struggling, and failing, to achieve results, assume there is something wrong with them. They believe that something very unique to themselves is preventing success. This is quite common, however, it is not true! While you are a beautiful and unique snowflake, you are not broken, and you aren't as different as you think. While a very small percentage of people do suffer from illnesses and health issues that make reaching health goals very difficult, they are a minority.

In my experience, I believe the problem is years and years of bad fad diets, bad information, and psychological self-bullying. The problem is years of built up "elephants" that get bigger and bigger with each year they go ignored.

4

What Is YOUR Elephant?

In my years of working with clients as a Personal Trainer and Integrative Nutrition Health Ccoach, I have found the *number one* obstacle to achieving fitness, diet, and weight loss success. It's the ELEPHANT IN THE ROOM!

The 'elephant in the room' is your psychological barrier to success. There are a few 'elephants' I want to discuss in this book. First, let's C my A (that's an abbreviation for the term "cover my a%@," in case you were wondering):

I am not a counselor, therapist, nor psychologist. This book is not trying to fix you. The goal of this book is to encourage you to start thinking more deeply about the *'whys'* of the things you do and don't do regarding your health. My hope is that you begin cleaning out your emotional cupboard and, if needed, seek professional help in order to work through your cupboard faster.

So, what is your 'elephant'?

The following 'elephants' are the psychological barriers I have noticed in myself, my friends, my family, and my clients over the years. Many people struggle with these issues. So, if you identify with one or all of them, there is nothing broken about you. Knowing is half the battle. Acknowledging what is in your emotional cupboard is the first step. Taking things out and cleaning things up is something for you to do in your own time, when you are ready.

Think of it like you're cleaning out the garage. You can probably move the small boxes, the bikes, and the knickknacks by yourself— these are smaller, lighter, and don't require help. These are the elephants you can address and fix on your own through some changing, learning, reading, and growing. However, you probably can't move the power saw by yourself, or the extra couch, or the broken fridge. These things are large, they are heavy, and you need help to move them. These are the 'elephants' I believe a therapist can help with.

When I started going to therapy, that's how I looked at it. I needed help moving my psychological refrigerators. A trained professional was the fastest and best way for me to do it. I wanted to be psychologically stronger and fitter, and I wanted results as quickly as possible. Therapy allowed me to get straight to the nitty-gritty. It allowed me to come out on the other side much faster than had I tried to go it alone. I am so, eternally thankful that I put my pride aside, (and this was a very difficult thing for me to do) and sought professional help. I can't, and don't want to, imagine where I'd still be if I hadn't.

Addressing 'elephants' can be a very difficult and emotional journey. I can tell you from personal experience that once you do clean out your cupboard, you will be so glad you did.

A friend of mine once equated every challenge in our life to a high fence. Our current situation being the side of the fence we are on and the fence being the challenge itself. We know what we have on this side of the fence where we currently are. We are familiar with it. It feels safe. We want to jump the high fence to something new and different, but we can't see over the fence to know what lies on the other side. So we are scared. What if we don't like it over there?

The fence is high; what if we fall as we try to climb it?

I can tell you this: there is a good chance you will fall while climbing the fence. We all slip and fall sometimes. So what? The worst thing that could happen is that you end up right back where you started, on your side of the fence. You already know what it is like on this side. As we said before, it's familiar and feels safe.

What if you don't like it on the other side of the fence? What if it is too scary or too different? Then, you can climb back over to where you began. It's that simple. Although, I don't think you'll want to do that.

I can also tell you this: once I climbed my first fence and faced my first psychological challenge, once I took that leap toward a better life, I didn't ever want to go back to where I began. I climbed my first fence and loved it. So, I climbed a second, then a third, and I'm still not done. I know that with each fence I climb, each 'elephant' that I address, I am happier and healthier than before. Not once have I wanted to climb back.

OK, so let's get started!

5

No Sugar Coating

Let's get a few things out in the open before we begin.

I don't sugarcoat things and I won't tip-toe around a point in order to save your feelings. I believe there has been too much of that going on, and that is part of the problem.

I am not going to tell anyone what size or weight they should be. I tell all my clients that when they feel their sexiest, they are at their perfect weight and size. For some, this is a size three; for others, it is a size fourteen, and everything below, between, and above.

My concern is for health! We have a very serious health epidemic going on here in the US. Heart disease, hypertension, fibromyalgia, atherosclerosis, diabetes, cancer, and all other degenerative diseases are depriving us and our loved ones of quality of life. In the words of the great Dr. Myron Wentz, "We are living too short, and dying too long."

I remember when I first became interested in health. I was very young, in middle school. I was the odd duck in high school and Junior College who was exercising, eating veggies, taking vitamins, etc. I remember people teasing me and joking, asking, "Why bother Gemma? Do you want to live forever?" Even then, my reply was "No, I don't want to live forever, but I'm sure going to do my best to not spend the last twenty years of my life in a bed, hooked up to a machine." This answer always stumped my harasser!

In the words of the great Dr. Myron Wentz, "People are living too short, and dying too long."

So know that my passion on this topic of the psychology of dieting and fitness is not about telling you what you should weigh or what size you should wear. That has nothing to do with me. That is a personal decision for you to make.

But I am concerned with your health.

Health, to me, means physical, psychological and spiritual health! They are all equally important.

I won't be delving into spiritual health here. But I do challenge you to find your spiritual truth.

What we will be discussing is the effect of your psychological health on your physical health.

So, what is the 'elephant in the room'?

The 'elephant in the room' is any psychological barrier to success that hinders you from reaching your diet, fitness, and weight loss goals.

Most people ignore their psychological issues, thinking they'll deal with them another day, sometime in the future. Then they continue to struggle with diet, struggle with fitness, and struggle with weight loss. They try and fail time and time again (which causes even more psychological barriers) without achieving success.

Here's a nugget for you:

If you keep doing what you're doing, you're going to keep getting what you're getting.

If you want something to change, you're going to have to change something.

It is THAT simple!

But it's hard work to deal with the psychological stuff! Issues may have been brushed aside and put in a metaphorical cupboard, collecting dust, for years on end. There may be years' worth of feelings of failure as fad diet after fad diet didn't work. Years' worth of feelings of guilt over hundreds, even thousands, of wasted dollars on gym memberships and fitness programs that went unused. Years' worth of feelings of defeat after failing again and again.

It is my goal with this book to shed some light on those dark corners of your mind where unaddressed feelings may be hiding. Let's pull them out into the light of day and dust them off once and for all.

6

Diets Don't Work

So you want to be healthier and lose weight?

Just eat less junk, eat more healthy stuff, and exercise every day!

Easy, right?

If it were that simple, then the diet and weight loss industry wouldn't be raking in $20 billion dollars annually.[ii] And the fitness industry wouldn't be netting $17.6 billion each year.[iii]

How many diets and programs have you tried?

One? Two? Five? Ten? Or more?

If you're like most Americans, you have jumped on the diet bandwagon several times a year, every year, for decades.

Let me share a little secret with you: Diets don't work!

If they did, we wouldn't have so many of them. We'd have one that works and we'd all be healthy with low body fat percentages. The end!

Research on dieting shows that diets have a detrimental effect on the dieter's self-esteem and on the body. Diets that deprive the body of food and calories result in the loss of lean muscle, which causes the body's metabolism to slow down.

Let's take a closer look at those two sentences.

1.) *"Research on dieting shows that diets have a detrimental effect on the dieter's self-esteem and on the body."*

A person who diets is most likely already in a state in which they have a lowered self-esteem and are unhappy with their body. They diet to '*fix*' these issues. However, research shows that body-image and self-esteem usually are worse after a diet. What do we do when we feel bad about ourselves? I don't know about you, but I eat! A lot! This, in turn, causes more weight-gain than I needed to lose in the first place. It's a vicious cycle of failure.

2.) *"Diets that deprive the body of food and calories result in the loss of lean muscle, which causes the body's metabolism to slow down."*

A higher metabolism means that your body is able to burn more calories all day long, even when not exercising. Metabolism and muscle mass are directly associated with each other. More muscle means higher metabolism. This is why athletes can eat so much without gaining body fat. Low-calorie or low-protein diets cause the body to lose muscle. Thus, the metabolism goes down. As soon as the dieter starts eating a healthy amount of food again they actually GAIN more weight than they needed to lose in the first place because the metabolism is lower. This makes future weight loss even more difficult. A few cycles of this and the metabolism is really low (eating right and exercising can increase the metabolism). In fact, the average results per diet today is not a weight loss, but a gain of seven pounds.[iv]

No wonder your self-esteem is shot, right?

Does this sound familiar?

If this sounds like you, then it's time to stop the train! Get off the diet roller coaster and start getting real.

It's time to address the 'elephant in the room'!

7

Overwhelmed, Confused, and Frustrated

It's very difficult to figure out what to eat and how to exercise when each new fad and program that comes along contradicts the last one. Also, it's confusing when the food industry takes advantage of our health concerns by advertising and marketing information that just isn't correct. I notice that many of my clients are confused, overwhelmed, and frustrated with this overload of conflicting information.

It IS overwhelming, confusing, and frustrating. That's why I'm here. It is my job to help my clients through all the confusion to the real, scientific-based information that gets results!

Typically, after only a few short weeks of working with me in my programs, my clients start to see results. When they tackle inner demons, learn to change, and learn to learn; confusion, frustration, and presumed brokenness make way for clarity. Mental walls come crashing down as truth is discovered.

There are many things to learn on the journey to health. Nutrition and exercise should be dynamic aspects of your life, ever evolving and growing. Don't just pick one thing and do it forever. As the body changes, along with life's demands, so should your diet and exercise regimen. Be prepared to continue learning for the rest of your life.

Did you get that? Did you absorb what you just read?

If you want to change your health and your body, then you must *LEARN, GROW, CHANGE*, and *ADAPT*. In order to *see* change, you must *create* change. What you have been doing has not been working, so you must learn a new way and implement it.

Read that paragraph a few times, then close your eyes and see yourself doing things differently. Visualize yourself eating healthy food, cooking healthy food, and buying healthy food. Imagine yourself exercising, and enjoying it. Make peace with the ideas of change, growth, and learning. You must do these things if you want results—REAL results.

8

Negative Self-Talk

The number one most debilitating thing I have noticed hindering people from achieving their fitness and weight loss goals is this:

The inner voice. The voice inside your head!

This is something I discuss in some of my fitness classes and seminars. I like to talk with my classes and "get real." I like to address this issue right there, in front of your face, while you are exposed in a room full of others. It's raw, it's hard, and it's real. I see the faces in class, the tears in the eyes, the realization that they have been guilty of this. I often cry myself. This one is huge and most common with women.

Let's take a break for a moment. I want to tell you a story.

My 6-year-old niece had been begging me to take her ice skating for months. She decided that she wanted to be an Olympic figure-skater when she grew up, and she needed to start training now if she was going to make it.

Finally, last winter, I took her to the skating rink and signed her up for a beginner lesson. She spent the entire day before her lesson picking out the perfect outfit for skating. It took her an hour to do her hair the morning of the lesson. She insisted on being completely ready for her first lesson, as if it were her actual Olympic tryout.

Putting on the rental skates before the lesson I thought she was going to just burst from sheer joy, happiness, and excitement. You could see her dreams coming true right before her very eyes. She was envisioning standing on that podium receiving the gold medal at the Olympics.

She was beyond elated.

I helped her to the ice and the lesson began.

Have you ever watched the Disney movie Bambi? There's a scene in the movie when Bambi discovers a frozen pond and tries to walk on it. He wobbles, slips, slides, and gets his legs all tangled. Go and find it on YouTube it if you haven't seen it.

Well, let's just say that if my niece had been as clumsy as Bambi, it would have been a huge improvement from her performance on the ice that day.

She was not an instant success on the ice.

After many falls and great frustration over being the only one in the lesson who couldn't get it together, my niece scrambled off the ice in tears. She came to me and declared that she "QUIT." That ice skating was *not* what she wanted to do anymore. She didn't really want to go to the Olympics anyway.

I knew I had to step in and help this poor kid out.

I sat her little 6-year-old self down, face-to-face, and told her to listen and listen hard. Then I said this to her:

"I had big hopes for you today. I really wanted you to be an instant success as an ice-skater. I love that you had a dream to be an Olympic figure skater—which would have been pretty awesome. But, you sucked ice out there. You were the WORST kid in the class. I've never seen ANYONE fall as much as you did. It was brutal to watch. I mean, I felt sorry for you. You just looked so pathetic out there. I think you've made the right decision to not pursue this ice skating dream. I think it's probably best for everyone involved. I wouldn't want to sit and watch as you suffer through agonizing lessons week after week anyway. And that poor instructor— I don't think he knew WHAT to do with you! You truly looked like a three-legged giraffe on roller skates. Let's go home and watch TV. After all, you're good at that at least!"

SAY WHAT!?!?!?!?!?!?!

Ok, ok, ok! Simmer down.

I don't have a niece! That was just a hypothetical story to prove a point.

If this were real life, I would have given the child a pep-talk. As grown-ups, we all know that it takes practice to become great at something. We understand that we're going to fall down a *lot* on our journey to greatness. We get that we are going to fail, but we have to pick ourselves backup and keep going. It takes time, dedication, spirit, and determination to become great at something. No child is going to put on ice skates and be instantly fantastic (unless they're a prodigy). However, with lessons and practice, she may just become an Olympic winner. We *know* this, *right*?

RIGHT?!

Then why, when we do not achieve instant results with fitness and diet, do we tell ourselves that we suck, that we are losers, that we are just fat and lazy and should just give up? Why do we expect to become instant experts overnight and not realize that these things take practice?

Think about this for a minute...

We know that in our careers, we will often fall and get back up over and over again before we reach our goals. We know that it takes time, practice, and patience to become great at something.

Yet, when it comes to eating healthy and exercising, we expect instant perfection.

I have clients who are tremendously successful doctors, entrepreneurs, lawyers, etc. who struggle with this very issue. They are able to apply logic in every area of their lives *except* when it comes to diet and exercise.

I have noticed that this is an issue with which *many* people struggle.

How can you be expected to be successful when that voice inside your head is telling you horrible, terrible things that break your spirit? What happens to children who are verbally abused? They have significant confidence, self-esteem, and love issues if not addressed with therapy. We know this, and yet many people verbally abuse themselves constantly.

How can you expect success when you do nothing to encourage yourself?

Why are you nastier to yourself than you are to your worst enemy? It's time to become your biggest supporter. You must be your own greatest fan. It's okay to tell yourself that *you rock*. There is nothing wrong with giving yourself credit and giving yourself pep-talks. It is not egotistical. It is not weird. It is a great way to reach success.

What does your inner voice tell you? Does it say, "You are amazing!" "You are beautiful!" "You are a lovely person with a great heart." "You're a hard worker and an asset to any organization." "You can do it, go for it!"? Or does your inner voice sound more like this, "You're an idiot." "You're fat and lazy." "Why would anyone want to date you?" "Hey Dummy, what are you thinking?" "You're never going to be in shape."?

If you picked the latter statements, then you are suffering from negative self-talk.

If negative self-talk is your elephant in the room, here is your assignment.

Get a rubber band, one of those rubber bracelets or a rubber bracelet and place it around your wrist. (I'll tell you what to do with it in a bit).

You are going to train your brain out of this very damaging bad habit. That's what it is—a bad habit. Negative self-talk is a habit, and habits can be broken with hard work and persistence. Acknowledging it is a powerful first step. Thich Nhat Hanh wrote in *A Blessing in Disguise - 39 Life Lessons from Today's Greatest Teachers,* "The moment we recognize any habit energy, it loses a little of its power." So, recognize any habit you have, and take away some of its power over you.

9

The Rubber Band
Conditioning Project

A few years ago, a friend of mine and I were talking. We were both students at West Virginia University; I was studying Exercise Physiology, and she was studying Sports Psychology. We loved discussing what we were learning about in our classes. She was a college athlete, so she offered a great perspective as both an athlete and as someone studying the psychology of sports performance. She taught me a few things I have used to help my clients ever since.

Athletes use the power of their brains to help them win. Mental toughness can be that one factor, that edge, which may be the difference between a win and a loss. This friend told me how her coach had told her to put a rubber band around her wrist. If she ever thought about losing, she was to snap the band against her wrist. Not enough to break the skin, but enough to elicit a little sting. If she ever envisioned a missed shot, a slip-up, or a losing score, she was to snap that band.

Why? To condition her brain to WIN!

Don't snap the band so hard that you actually injure yourself. Just a little snap and a mild sting, okay?

You see, when it comes to mental conditioning, we're not much more complex than a rat being trained in a maze. In psychological conditioning experiments, a rat will receive an electrical shock if they go the wrong way in a maze or do something the researchers do not want the rats to do. In very little time, the rat becomes 'conditioned' to *not* do the thing that causes a shock. They are trained to perform the task desired by the researchers.

Our brains work the same way. The band snap is like that shock. We can train our brains out of bad habits. So, by snapping that band when thinking about losing, the brain gets trained. After a time, the brain equates thinking about losing with pain and then doesn't think about losing anymore for fear of feeling pain.

This works for negative self-talk, too. Every time you think anything negative about yourself, I want you to snap the rubber band. Do this every time until you have trained your brain out of this bad habit.

(I reiterate—do not harm yourself in this practice. You should not leave marks behind on your body from the band snap. It should be a slight, very minor sting. If you physically harm yourself, then we can't be friends anymore. Got it?!)

EXTRA CREDIT

I don't want you to stop there. I would like you to go for extra credit. Each time you snap the band after thinking something negative about yourself, I would like you to think three *good* things about yourself. This may be awkward at first. Sadly, we are often better at pointing out our flaws than our strengths. Still, keep at it. Practice makes perfect.

You may have to get a little silly with this extra credit challenge at first. The three good things you say about yourself might be, "I am a princess," "Everyone wants to be my friend." And "I am a good driver." No matter how silly you feel—keep doing it.

In fact, the very fact that you feel silly listing positive things about yourself is proof that you desperately need to do this exercise.

In time, you will get better at complimenting yourself and you will begin to notice your many great attributes. "Hey! I have a great butt," or, "Hey! I'm an amazing friend," or, "Hey! My eyes are gorgeous!"

The more you do this, the more you will notice the good things about *you*.

BONUS:

The rubber band practice can work for you in other scenarios, too. When faced with unhealthy treats that you don't want to eat, you can snap the rubber band and train your brain out of your craving for junk.

10

You've Got the Power
(of Visualization)

My friend studying sports psychology (the one I talked about in the last chapter) also told me about a study she was reading in school. In the study, researchers had a team of collegiate basketball players shoot free throws. Results were recorded, and the percentage of successful shots was calculated. The team was then divided in half, and each group was sent into separate rooms. The first group was told to close their eyes and visualize shooting the basketball and making it into the basket every single time. They could not imagine missing. The second group was told to close their eyes and visualize missing the basket every single time they shot the ball. After a short period of time, the groups went back out onto the court and shot free throws again. Averages for each group were recorded.

As you may have guessed, the first group, the group that visualized making every shot, increased their percentage of successful free throws. The percentage for the second group, on the other hand, decreased significantly.

By just the power of thought, performance was improved or hindered. This is how powerful the mind is. You can train your brain to be your best ally or your biggest adversary. Since you'll have your mind for your whole life (unless you lose it), think carefully about how you train it.

Negative self-talk can be a lot more damaging than you may have realized. It's time to lift up yourself and others, and start using that powerful coconut of yours in order to achieve great success in fitness, weight loss, and beyond!

11

Cement Shoes

Deciding to start living a healthier lifestyle is an easy decision. Actually doing it, however, is something else. The inner battles (as we've been discussing) are hard enough to overcome. Surrounding yourself with people who will support you in your efforts can make a huge difference.

However, some people can drag you down. They will try to sabotage you, every step of the way.

"You're losing too much weight." "You look sick"." Are you really going to eat that rabbit food?" "Come on, eat a piece of cake—it won't kill you." "You're going to the gym, again?" "I think you have an obsession!" "You're no fun anymore." "You know you won't keep this up." The list of things I've heard goes on and on.

While you're trying to swim your way to a healthier life, these people can be the cement shoes that attempt to drag you down. They just pull you under no matter how hard you try. You must arm yourself for battle when dealing with these types of people.

A client of mine, Amber, had a very difficult time with this one. Amber came to my early morning Sunrise Shred exercise group three times a week, she kept a food journal, and ate a clean, well balanced meals every three to four hours throughout the day. She was taking her USANA Essentials, multi-vitamin and multi-mineral, twice a day. She was getting stronger, leaner, healthier, and fitter. She had more energy, was sleeping better, and her skin was clearer. Her whole life was improving. Except when it came to her "friends."

Amber's friends would constantly make negative comments about her new healthy lifestyle. They would say all the things listed above, and worse. It caused her so much stress. She was truly hurt by their words. After our morning workouts we would spend a lot of time together discussing how to deal with these "haters" and arming her for the day ahead.

Negative comments from strangers are one thing, but negative comments from those who should be your biggest supporters is a horse of a different color. They hurt so much more.

It is difficult enough to go to a birthday party and not eat the cake. It is practically impossible to resist when your "friends" are shoving it in your face trying to talk you into taking "just a bite."

It's utterly demoralizing to finally reach a milestone goal in your journey, to feel so amazing about it, only to be told by a "friend" that you're obsessed and looking ill.

These people are called *cement shoes.*

If this is your 'elephant', then you need to know this very important fact:

These comments from your 'cement shoes' are *never* a reflection of you. It is *always* a reflection on *them.*

When you set a goal and reach it right before someone's eyes, you are a big reminder to them that it *can* be done, and that they *could* do it too. Yet they aren't doing anything at all!

If you fail, then, "There you go! See, that's why I don't bother. Everyone fails when they try to get healthy. Just look at my friend who failed." They can hide behind your failure. However, your success is a huge slap in their face that it is possible, but they are choosing not to make changes of their own.

So, arm yourself now for this 'elephant'.

First, try to distance yourself from the Negative Nellies out there. Who needs to be surrounded by Rodney Rain Clouds anyway?

Second, realistically, you can't get rid of people you love just because they're a little unsupportive, so try talking to those closest to you *before* you embark on your journey to better health. Explain to them what your goals are. Share with them how important this is to you. Let them off the hook, and reassure them that you will not judge them if they eat cake in front of you, just ask them to not offer any to you. Ask for their help and support. Let them know how they can help and support you. Explaining to loved ones that you don't want them to offer you junk or bring you your favorite chocolate when they visit may sound simple, but people have a hard time changing habits. Don't get upset if you have to ask a thousand times.

Third, prepare yourself. Be such a loud and effective cheerleader for yourself that the negative comments from others won't derail you.

Be prepared for those people in your life who will try to drag you down like cement shoes. Remind yourself every day that this is *their* issue, not yours. Prepare a number of power-packed responses.

For example, if a "cement shoe" says, "Come on, just eat a piece of cake, for crying out loud. This is getting ridiculous." One response could be, "Thanks for the offer, but I don't want the cake. I could eat it if I wanted to. But I don't *want* it. I'm really enjoying my new way of eating, so quit getting on my case. I don't get on your case for eating the cake."

Think of a number of possible retorts to those comments from cement shoes. Arm yourself for battle against those who stand to drag you down and away from your goals.

Stop and think:

If people you love and respect start expressing concern for your weight loss and start throwing around terms like "eating disorder" or "anorexia", I would like you to take these seriously. Healthy lifestyles can sometimes get a little out of hand and we don't always see ourselves the way we really are. So, if you hear these comments, consider seeing a medical professional to check your weight and body fat. If you are fine, then you'll have medical proof of it, and you can silence your critics from saying anything more on the issue. However, if you are getting too thin then seeking that help as early as possible is the best way to get healthy the fastest.

BONUS:

Here are some *extremely* important things you need to know when you decide to make healthier choices:

1.) Don't ever complain about your new healthy choices. Don't complain about the salad you're eating. Don't complain about going to the gym. Don't complain about switching to whole grains, etc.

    a. Complaining invites the haters to jump and start trash-talking your new regime, too. Don't get them started and don't give them any ammo.

    b. Complaining affects your mental resolve to make changes. You don't *have* to eat a salad. You're a grown person who can make their own decisions. You can eat whatever the heck you like. You can eat the double cheeseburger with fries. But you don't want to. You are *choosing* to eat a salad for a trillion reasons (list them ten times a day if you need to in order to stay motivated). Healthy choices are not a punishment. Making them so will surely lead to failure.

2.) While you are with friends and faced with unhealthy treats, don't *ever* say, "I'm on a diet," "I can't eat that," "That's not on my program," "There's too much fat in that," or *"Oh mah gawd!* I can't eat that; it has too many carbs."

   a. Comments like this can make those eating the "treat" feel bad about themselves, and that's not nice, so don't do it.

   b. You open up a can of worms for everyone in your presence to try and convince you to "cheat" and eat the treat. Don't put yourself in that situation. It's way too difficult to fight.

3.) What you DO say (I don't advocate fibbing, but I say it's okay in these cases):

   a. "No thanks, I don't want any."

   b. "No thanks, I don't like that."

   c. "No thanks, I'm full."

   d. And, the clincher…"No thanks, I'm allergic."

   e. This is where you *live* when changing your eating habits. THE END. Don't veer from these given options. Capiche?

You're welcome!

12

It's Not Me; It's You

My friend Kelly shared her 'elephant' with me:

"I have found that sometimes the reactions of people you love to the changes you make in your life can be scary. All sorts of emotions can come up for them and for you, and it can be easy to fall into old habits...because you want your relationships to stay the same. But change is often necessary, and if you can learn to demonstrate to others how better health can mean a better life, hopefully you can come out on the other side. People get used to the "old" you and the old dynamics."

This one overlaps with 'cement shoes' a little, but I wanted to address it separately.

As I said at the beginning of this book, it's easy to change yourself but practically impossible to change others. Sometimes our healthful changes bring unwilling loved ones kicking and screaming into our new healthy lives.

I'll share a personal example to explain:

I live in the United States now but was born in Great Britain. I've lived in the US since I was 9 years old. If any of you know a Brit, you know about our national affinity for Cadbury's chocolate. It's a cultural necessity that cannot be understood by a non-Brit.

When we first moved to the US, our British family members would visit often and bring with them bags and bags of English chocolate. I think it was what my parents bartered in exchange for room and board at our house.

I cannot resist English chocolate. I once sat on the couch and ate seventeen chocolate bars in one sitting, and would have eaten more had I not run out; I would practically inhale the yummy treats from across the pond.

I had no willpower against this chocolate (I still don't).

As I grew older and started eating healthier, I learned that I could not keep treats in the house, or else I would inhale them. However, my family members continued to bring and send me tons of English chocolate. It was how they showed me love and that they were thinking of me. I asked them, repeatedly, to not bring me chocolate anymore or to just bring me one chocolate bar. Yet nothing changed; they would bring bags of it. And, I couldn't resist it.

I asked for things to change for years with no results. Finally, I knew I had to take drastic measures if I wanted to stop this family habit.

Then one day my Aunty brought me a bag full of chocolate bars, after I asked her to only bring me one bar. I ate one and then threw all the others in the trash (it pained me to do so). She saw them all in the garbage and got upset. I apologized, and explained to her that I couldn't have treats in the house or I would eat them. I told her about my efforts to eat healthier. She got upset and told the whole family what I had done, and how rude I was. She got over it a few days later, but no one has brought or sent me bags of chocolate since. MISSION ACCOMPLISHED. I now get ONE chocolate bar, and that's all I want and need.

It took years of begging and then a drastic action to get my family to hear my plea. But, I finally won the battle.

Changing others is difficult!

This 'elephant' affects a lot of couples and parents who adopt new, healthier lifestyles. Friday night family night with pizza and ice cream will be a challenge to the healthy eater. I don't suggest changing rituals abruptly as you'll face an angry mob. Rather, prepare for them and have a salad and fresh fruit instead. Over time you can start offering salad with pizza and fruit with ice cream for the rest of the family. Let them choose to try them. Don't force anyone into your new lifestyle. Just be prepared for this type of thing.

Do you have a hobby of playing video games with your loved one? Is it your usual day-long activity on the weekends? Then consider getting up early and, going to the gym first. You can get your workout in before beginning your day of video games.

Ease your loved ones into these changes. Tell them, "Honey, I think I may start getting up an hour earlier on Saturday mornings to go to the gym before we hang out. I always feel better after the gym. Is that okay with you?" Hopefully they'll say yes; if not now, then, eventually. Also, it helps to do something nice for them for a few weeks after making the change, just to butter them up a bit.

Communication is key; don't give up. People may test your resolve. It may just take time for others to realize that you mean business, that things are changing and they'd better get on board. Be patient and don't give up!

13

Trapped in a Fat Suit

Change can be very difficult, especially when it comes to losing weight. We get used to who we are, how people treat us, our patterns, habits, and reactions to things. Losing weight comes with a lot more than a change in pant size.

If you have been heavy for a large part of your life, you have built your realities, relationships, hobbies, and personality around being heavy.

Having beers and cheese fries every weekend with the boys, drinking wine and eating brownies on girls night, getting ice cream with the kids, pizza night, Chinese take-out, playing video games or watching movies during all your free time...these are all things that become part of your life in a very emotional way.

Perhaps you have surrounded yourself with heavy friends who share all these habits with you. Maybe you like to crack on skinny people or even make jokes about yourself being fat or skipping the gym again. There's even a cartoon I've seen circulating on social media that says, "I missed the gym again today. That's 10 years in a row."

My friend Kristy shared her elephant in the room with me:

"I took the label of "fat"' and made it a part of my personality. It was my "persona". I was the fat chick. It was what made me different from most of my friends, but I had (to the outside world) a healthy confidence about myself, while inwardly I was EXTREMELY insecure. Without my "fat girl" persona, I had no jokes I could crack on myself, nothing to talk about, and nothing special about me (or so I thought for a long time). I was scared to let it go, because then, who was I? I was too afraid to find out or let others find out just in case I wasn't anyone special."

Kristy brings up such a great point. She used her weight as a way to make jokes. She made people laugh by putting herself at the butt of those jokes. This ties into the negative self-talk that we just discussed (many of these elephants overlap). It is damaging on many levels. Change has so many layers. It's something to consider and prepare yourself for before you start your journey to health.

What areas of your life have you tied to your lack of health or fitness? Will your friends try to talk you out of your goals? What areas and relationships in your life will have to change as you change? What rituals or hobbies revolve around unhealthy habits? These are all things that need to be addressed *before* you attempt to reach your goals. If you ignore these issues, they'll eventually come back and smack you square in the face, possibly derailing you from success.

I struggled with my weight for many years. I yo-yoed up and down for seventeen years. I was always at the gym, but I was a little rounder than everyone else. I exercised like a fiend, but I didn't know how to eat.

I had an 'elephant in my room'. Mine was an aversion to sexual attention. You know the look you get when someone thinks you look good? They give you the down-and-up glance as they scan you from head to toe? I refer to it as "the once-over." I hated that look. And, I do mean HATED. It made my skin crawl. I wanted to crawl into a hole and disappear when it happened to me.

Each time I would start to eat right and lose weight, someone would, inevitably, give me the once-over. I would be disgusted and feel so uncomfortable that I would go home and EAT! I hated that attention so much that it caused me to self-sabotage. I would eat to gain my weight back to avoid that look.

After years of doing this I was finally able to identify it as an 'elephant'. It was a barrier to my goals. I knew that I wanted to look like a fitness professional. I wanted to look like I had been in the gym for hours a day and that I taught group fitness and was a personal trainer. I had to look my elephant square in the eye. I decided that my goal to look like a fitness professional and be my own advertising was more important than those few moments of feeling uncomfortable. I told myself that it was okay for people to look at my body and admire my hard work. I realized that people are going to have sexual thoughts about me no matter what I look like. That had nothing to do with me. I had to let it go and move forward to my goals.

It didn't happen right away. Rather, it was a slow journey of acceptance. However, I am now, thankfully, over that 'elephant'.

Being trapped in a fat suit can go very deep and get very serious. I have had clients who were victims of assault and rape when they were thinner. In order to protect themselves from such a terrible crime happening again, they wear a fat suit so as not to be sexually appealing. This is definitely something that should be addressed with a professional counselor, but it can be repaired, if you get help and do the work. Don't ignore these things as they just get bigger and bigger the longer they sit in your cupboard. I can tell you, from seeing these clients achieve great success, you too can address and conquer issues such as these, with help. ☺

14

Guess I'll Go Eat Worms

Remember that little song, "Nobody likes me; everybody hates me. I guess I'll go eat worms?" Well, that song is the inspiration for the title of this chapter.

For some people, their elephant is a perceived lack of support from others.

I have heard people complain to me that they can't lose weight because there isn't anyone to help them. No one will go on the diet with them. No one will wake them up to go to the gym. No one will walk with them. No one will cook them healthy food, etc.

This is a tricky one because it has many layers to it. Why must you have someone else with you on your journey to health and weight loss? Why don't you feel that you alone can accomplish your goals? In what other areas of your life are you not reaching your potential due to the lack of a posse at your side?

If this is your 'elephant', you may have tried oodles of programs and diets with friends who said they would do them with you; however, as soon as they flake, you quit too. It's time to start believing that you do not need a buddy to hold your hand on your journey. You alone are strong enough, disciplined enough, motivated enough, and able enough to do it alone. You are enough.

Get your rubber band on, and train that brain of yours to believe that you can do it alone.

Sure, it's nice to have a buddy by your side for the weight loss ride. It's great to meet a friend at the gym for a class, but they are not your reason for making healthy choices. You are.

Make a list of all the reasons you are exercising and/or eating healthy. Remind yourself of these reasons multiple times a day. Let these reasons be enough motivation to keep you on track even if no one in your life is supporting you to do so. Read through the earlier chapters and build yourself up and train your brain so that you don't need others to justify your goals.

YOU are enough!

15

The Blame Game, Yawn!

I can't lose weight because my mom cooks, and she makes really unhealthy things.
I can't exercise because it hurts my ankle.
I can't eat vegetables because I don't know how to cook them.
I can't exercise because I can't afford a gym membership.
I can't stick to a diet because my mother didn't feed me healthy food when I was a child.

I have heard some doozy excuses for why people can't get healthy.

There isn't an excuse that doesn't make me yawn! No matter how creative the reason, they are all the same thing: an excuse.

Someone once said, "If you really want something, you'll find a way. If you really don't, you'll find an excuse."

There is always an excuse not to go to the gym. *The dishes need to be done, the dog needs his teeth brushed, I'm tired, I have to visit my neighbor.* There are always good excuses for skipping a workout. *I'm tired and need more rest. I think I overdid it last time so I should rest today. I missed the class I like, so I just won't go.* Etc.

There has to come a point when your desire for change is stronger than any excuse you can throw at it.

In *Become A Better You: 7 Keys to Improving Your Life Every Day* by Joel Osteen, I read this, "Take responsibility for your own actions. You may have experienced some unfair things in the past that have made life more difficult for you, but your attitude should be, 'I'm not going to sit around and moan and complain about how I was raised or about how somebody mistreated me. No, this is the life God gave me, and I'm going to make the most of it. I'm going to make good choices starting today.'"

I've mentioned this already: make a list of all the reasons you do want to eat healthy, and all the reasons you do want to exercise. Keep this list with you, post it up at work, and put it where you can see it and be reminded of it.

I find quotes to be extremely motivating at those times when I just don't want to make the right choice. I used to have a terrible time getting up in the morning for a workout (Who am I kidding? I still do). I would create a great excuse in my head to justify staying under my warm covers and falling back asleep. Then I saw a great commercial—I think it was for Nike. A mother woke up when it was still dark, checked on her sleeping husband and kids, and then went out for a jog. As she reached the top of a hill, the sun was rising before her and she smiled with utter satisfaction. The voice on the commercial said, "I sacrifice sleep for sunrises."

That commercial has stuck with me for years. The beauty of that sunrise was greater than that extra 20   minutes of sleep. Repeating that saying in my head has gott   ut of bed for a workout more times than I can co

Find your   gs, etc. Just find some   you from reaching you.

Excuses are old   ve and stop using them.

16

Grieving Isn't Just for after Death

*Disclaimer: The grief of losing a loved one is devastating. I am not, in any way, discounting that grief. I only aim to acknowledge that we can grieve many types of losses.

Grief is a very powerful thing. Grief is typically associated with the loss of a loved one, but grief can be felt after any loss.

Dictionary.com defines grief in this way:

Keen mental suffering or distress over affliction or loss; sharp sorrow; painful regret.

Grief isn't only felt after a death. Grief is a suffering after any significant loss, and *"Significant"* is a relative term. You cannot judge another's loss, no matter its magnitude. Feelings of grief are real for the person feeling them and must be dealt with in a healthy manner.

Grief may be felt over the loss of the life you had planned. For example, an injury which prevents you from continuing with your favorite fitness class may cause grief over the loss of doing what you loved. Grief can come from learning you cannot have any more children when you planned on having a house full of kids—this grief is for the loss of your dream family. People may suffer the loss of freedom and independence after learning that a disease will change the way they live their life.

Grief may come after any sort of loss.

However, when grief is felt for something other than the loss of a life, these feelings are sometimes confused, subdued, ignored, or suppressed. Since no one passed away, we don't always associate our feelings as grief.

I've talked with clients who felt guilty for being angry over a loss that doesn't involve a death. Yet, when we learn about grief, we learn that there are distinct stages to grief—*all* grief.

1. Shock and Denial
2. Pain and Guilt
3. Anger and Bargaining
4. Depression, Reflection, Loneliness
5. The Upward Turn
6. Reconstruction and Working Through
7. Acceptance and Hope

Each of these stages must occur in their own time. You cannot rush a stage of grief. Some may last a long time; some don't last long at all. But they must all occur for healing to truly happen.

I coach clients all over the world to help them with better nutrition, weight loss, lifestyle changes, and more. I recently spoke with a client who was upset about her size and wanted to lose weight. For several weeks we discussed her goals and her obstacles, but she just didn't seem ready to take the plunge and actually start incorporating changes.

One day, this client revealed to me she had recently learned she was unable to have any more children. Although she has one amazing child, she always dreamed of having a big family. Since receiving this sad news, she had not been able to find the focus to make healthy changes in her life and, therefore, had been gaining weight. She confessed to feeling angry and bitter, which in turn made her feel guilty. This was not the kind of person she thought she was.

This lovely soul received news which devastated the dream of a family that she held her whole life. On top of this loss, she added guilt over the feelings she was experiencing that are typical of grief.

I pointed out that she was grieving this loss and that anger and bitterness are one of the stages of grief. These feelings are normal and acceptable and must be felt fully, not buried and denied, if true healing is to occur. Recognizing grief is the first step in the healing process.

I have coached many clients who have suffered injuries which result in major lifestyle changes. A bulging disc, vertebral damage, loss of limb, paralysis, etc., each of these come with a long list of things the person can no longer do. Sometimes these clients have to cease participating in activities they have done for a lifetime, activities that bring them great joy and include their friends and social life, etc. For example, if an avid runner, who is in a running club and attends the group's social events and travels with other running friends to compete in marathons is told she can no longer run, she will experience major loss in multiple areas of her life. This loss must be grieved. The stages of grief must occur, and it's okay to feel them all. Shock, guilt, anger, loneliness, etc. —*all* of them are normal and okay.

I have also coached clients who received a diagnosis of a life-changing disease, such as autoimmune diseases, muscular degenerative diseases, chronic fatigue, digestive diseases, etc. With these diseases comes a significant change in lifestyle. Working all day *and* going to the gym *and* making a healthy dinner *and* spending time with family becomes impossible for someone with decreased energy and fatigue. For these people, it's a challenge just to get out of bed and get to work, let alone adding enjoyable activities to the day. People with digestive illnesses are slaves to their tummies and must adjust their entire schedule based on how their gut reacts to food that day. These illnesses come with a loss of the freedom of a life without disease. That loss results in grief. And that grief is normal, healthy, and acceptable.

We don't often acknowledge that these types of losses cause grief therefore we tend to bury our feelings and feel even guiltier for feeling them.

So, what to do? Acknowledging that there has been a loss and that you must grieve is the first step. Some grief can be dealt with on your own; however, sometimes we need a little help. Seeking counseling for grief and loss is not only acceptable but extremely helpful. It can aid you in healing faster than doing it alone. Don't be ashamed to seek out grief counseling for loss that doesn't involve loss of life.

If you have a loved one who is experiencing grief, be patient and accepting. You cannot judge another's feelings, ever. If someone feels grief, that grief is real, no matter what your opinion on the matter may be. To you it may not be a big deal that your sister can't have more kids; you don't want kids anyway, so this isn't as emotionally charged for you. Nonetheless, those feelings your sister is experiencing are very real and should be respected. You may be confused as to why your wife is so sad she can't run any more. She always complained about training for those marathons anyway. Besides now you can do more stuff together, so what's the big deal? These may be your feelings, but your wife has lost some large parts of her life that made her happy and contributed to her identity. Acknowledge and accept her losses. Don't ever try to minimize them.

Support your loved ones through their journeys and their feelings. You can't change how they feel and you can't fix it for them. All you can do is love and support them during a time they need it most.

If you are the one going through this, know that you are not broken and that your feelings are okay. It is very important that you deal with these feelings and experience each of the stages of grief if you are to heal. Trying to lose weight or focus on any new goals while experiencing feelings of grief can be extremely difficult. If grief is your 'elephant in the room', be patient with yourself as you travel through the seven stages.

So, identify the fact you have experienced a loss, understand the stages of grief and accept them, seek help even if you feel silly, and do your best every day. That's all anyone can do.

17

Moving the Couch (Getting Help)

I am not a therapist nor a counselor. I do not have a Psychology degree. However, I can challenge you to take your issues out of the cupboard, dust them off, and fix them.

I am a huge supporter of seeking professional help. I spent two years in therapy battling my own demons. My counselor helped me clean out my emotional cupboard a lot better and faster than I could have done on my own. I still need to go back and clean out my emotional attic and pantry, but I am not ready yet.

Seeking help does not make you weak. I used to think therapy was for weak people, and that I was strong enough to deal with things on my own. Then I hit a low that had me considering suicide. I was alone and overwhelmed. I realized that if I tried to get better on my own, it would take a very long time. I needed help. Going to therapy was the best thing I ever did. I spent one hour a week for almost two years with my therapist, working to clean out my emotional cupboard. I am a happier, healthier, nicer, more balanced person because of it. Admitting that I needed help and seeking it was the best thing I ever did.

I wouldn't be who I am today, where I am today, without those two years of counseling. (Thank you, Melanie, wherever you are!)

So don't let pride or shame prevent you from seeking help. Please, be brave enough to make that help a priority and seek it out.

18

That's a Wrap

So, there you have it—a number of 'elephants' I have experienced in my life and the lives of my clients and friends over the years. These are the most common issues, but these are not the only 'elephants' that you may be experiencing.

I truly hope that this book has challenged you to figure out what your 'elephant' is and to begin the task of pulling it out of your cupboard, cleaning it up, and getting rid of it.

Bottom line: if you have been yo-yo-ing for years with weight and health, trying every new fad diet and fitness trend but not achieving your goals, perhaps it's time to look under the hood and get to the bottom of things. Find your *why,* and the world of results will open up to you.

I'd love to hear from you. What is your 'elephant'? Did this book help you?

What steps do you think you are ready to take to clean out your own emotional closet?

Please share your thoughts and reviews of my book on Amazon and social media.

You can find me on social media and online:

Web:www. GemmaRayneFountain

Facebook: Gemma Rayne Fountain

Twitter: FitnessByGemma

Web: www.GemmaRayneFountain.USANA.com for all your nutrition, weight loss and skin care needs. Feel free to contact me for a free consultation to determine your supplement needs.

References

i) Elephant in the room. (2015, April 13). In *Wikipedia, The Free Encyclopedia*. Retrieved 04:31, April 20, 2015, from http://en.wikipedia.org/w/index.php?title=Elephant_in_the_room&oldid=656289034

ii) 100 Million Dieters, $20 Billion: The Weight Loss Industry by the Numbers. (2012, May 8). In *ABC News*. Retrieved 12:37, April 20, 2015, from http://abcnews.go.com/Health/100-million-dieters-20-billion-weight-loss-industry/story?id=16297197

iii) Lies of the Health and Fitness Industry Exposed. (2007, December 10). Pepin-Donat, Craig. In *Natural News: Natural Health News & Self Reliance*. Retrieved 12:40, April 20, 2015, from http://www.naturalnews.com/022358_health_fitness_industry.html

iv) How Diets Decrease Your Self-Esteem and Not Your Size. (2011, August 18). In *Adios Barbie: The Body Image Site for Every Body*. Retrieved 12:43, April 20, 2015, from http://www. adiosbarbie.com/2011/08/how-diets-decrease-your-self-esteem-and-not-your-size/

Acknowledgements

T hank you to all my clients I've worked with over the years. You have each taught me something and have helped contribute to the pages of this book.

To my mom for babysitting my children while I wrote and for all your support always. My husband for supporting this labor of love, and for loving me just as I am. To my kids for being the most amazing gifts from God, and the best things that have ever happened to me. To my dad for all your generous help this past few years. To Katy Kirby for editing so amazingly. To Chris Lopez for all your support and knowledge that you shared in this process. To Mike Watts for your time and shared knowledge that helped me stop stalling and make this happen. To Joel Cocker for being a catalyst. For Kevin Swango for an amazing book cover. To Sara Armistead for taking this project and making it so much greater than I ever could have envisioned myself. To the clients and friends who helped contribute to the content of this book. And for anyone who buys this, my first book. I hope it helps.

* About my dedication: Mrs. Anne Quarles was my 9th grade English Teacher. She took time to let me, a troubled teen, know that I was important and special. Her kind words and attention helped me to off a very self-destructive life path. I said then that I would dedicate my first book to her, so I did. Never underestimate the power of your love and attention, it can change lives.

22859830R00051

Made in the USA
San Bernardino, CA
17 January 2019